Born Strong Born Healthy

Frank V. Giulepp

Born Strong

Born Healthy

Francisco V. Giulepp

Copyright © Frank V. Giulepp

As always, the advice of a competent legal, tax, accounting or other professional should be sought. The author and publisher do not warrant the performance, effectiveness or applicability of any sites listed or linked to in this ebook. All links are for information purposes only and are not warranted for content, accuracy or any other implied or explicit purpose.

Table Of Contents

Introduction

On the off chance that you think, or know, that you are pregnant, we trust you have just visited your doctor!

Assuming that you have validated your intuitions and this is your first youngster, or that you wish to care more for yourself during pregnancy than you did during your different pregnancies; you have gone to the correct spot!

We will likely give all of you the data you should think about your wellbeing and the soundness of your unborn youngster during your pregnancy.

To do that, we trust it is significant for you to get pregnancy, and what is befalling your body as your child creates and approaches term.

Along these lines, all the data we give you about dealing with yourself will be explained with data about what is befalling your body and why it is critical to follow the proposals we offer you and the suggestions and guidance of your doctor.

To begin with, and chief, it is essential to counsel a doctor and to jump on a timetable of visits and testing to oblige each phase of your pregnancy.

In the event that you are sound and anticipate an ordinary pregnancy, you have a few choices for medicinal services during your pregnancy:

Obstetrician/Gynecologist (OB/GYN) – these doctors have a claim to fame in pregnancy and ladies' wellbeing.

Family General Practitioner or Internist – doctors who give standard clinical consideration to all people and at times will give obstetrical consideration.

Despite the fact that, misbehavior protection for this kind of clinical consideration has pointedly expanded, so much of the time, general specialists (GPs) and internists no longer conveyance infants, or treat ladies during the pregnancy term.

Along these lines, a considerable lot of these doctors will no longer think about a pregnant lady, yet rather will allude you to an OB/GYN.

Nurse/Midwives – these social insurance experts have some expertise in ladies' wellbeing and finish a pregnant mother pre-birth care, and work and conveyance.

At the point when you go to the doctor, she will check your weight, your circulatory strain and your midsection, check your infant's heartbeat, and ordinarily do a pelvic test.

A few ladies are awkward with these kinds of close tests and they do take some becoming acclimated to, on the off chance that you are not acquainted with yearly OB/GYN tests and pap spreads.

Be that as it may, these tests ARE imperative to your wellbeing and to the soundness of your infant.

Try not to miss arrangements, and don't accept all is well since you don't feel you have any side effects or issues. Let your medicinal services proficient do her/his activity!

Recall that once you realize you are pregnant, it is essential to deal with yourself.

You will get loads of guidance from everybody – even outsiders – about what you ought to do and what you ought NOT do.

It is essential to be instructed and educated, particularly if this is your first infant, so you feel certain that you realize what you are doing.

Else, you are probably going to be blown in the breeze as individuals offer clashing guidance, and you will feel dissipated and dubious.

Before we plunge into the subtleties of this book, we figured you may jump at the chance to make note of this site connect.

As you converse with your medicinal services proficient, you are probably going to hear a few words you have not heard previously.

Obviously, you ought to consistently request that your doctor clarify what you don't comprehend.

So let's begin this journey on how you can keep your baby strong and health during your pregnancy!.

One Effective Way to Ensure Pregnancy

From the early ages up to the contemporary occasions, fruitlessness is a difficult that consistently proceeds people everything being equal. Fruitlessness is a clinical and social worry that day break on nearly everyone paying little mind to the financial and social statuses, age, religion, shading, and race. Most definitely, fruitlessness is a sickness that influences the regenerative framework. Barrenness on both of the gatherings can make a serious injury both the mental and passionate well-creatures of both the male and the female accomplice.

Couples feel all the more joyful when the updates on pregnancy hits them. They feel practically complete by the minor idea that their dearest kid is in transit. The spouses to some degree become more cautious and all the more wanting to their wives. Then again, the eager moms are more wellbeing cognizant as they would like to make sure about that their child will be solid. The critical point in time presently lies in the couple's ability to consider. The two accomplices may appear to be typical and wellbeing savvy. However, there are as yet a great many situations when ripeness is by all accounts far close enough for a lot of wedded people.

A few ladies are honored with the endowment of getting pregnant problem free while there are the individuals who face injuries and significantly different troubles to consider. Ladies who don't effectively get pregnant must face the way that there are a ton of elements which may realize a trouble in their richness. Among the numerous reasons are one's state of being, age, and stress.

Is it accurate to say that you are encountering different troubles in getting pregnant? Have you attempted all strategies yet at the same time your endeavors are in vain? It might have been quite a while since you've had a go at imagining yet then there is no positive outcome that welcomes both of you. Presently you should deal with understanding reality that ladies are for the most part extraordinary. Be that as it may, to make things simple for you, the clinical society makes accessible the essential devices for you to take the fruitfulness test.

Kinds of Fertility Test

The richness test permits you to realize the very explanation concerning why you think that its difficult to get pregnant. You may counsel your most confided in richness authority for this issue.

The Hormone Testing. Different blood tests taken in various occasions are required for the hormone testing. The test is mostly for the discovery of the typical creation of hormone. The test henceforth assesses the amount of progesterone you have and on the off chance that you will have the option to continue a pregnancy. One of the blood tests done is to check your prolactin level. The hormone creates the bosom milk. Another test is to look at how your thyroid capacities.

The Ovulation Test. For this procedure, your gynecologist will be investigating the normality of your menstrual cycle. The instrument to be utilized is known as the ovulation expectation unit.

The Chlamydia and Gonorrhea Cultures. This test is acted so as to distinguish the conceivable nearness of these infections which are potential reasons for barrenness. They can be forestalled yet then its discovery is troublesome.

The Sperm Analysis. The test is directed to your accomplice to see the quality and check of the sperm.

The ripeness test is one way which enables your doctor to identify where the difficult falsehoods. Getting pregnant might be conceivable when the misstep in your body framework is remedied.

The most effective method to Use a Pregnancy Test

The topic of whether you are pregnant is regularly one of the most energizing, on edge, and upsetting inquiries that influence your wellbeing, yet your life. There are various sorts of pregnancy tests available or accessible through your essential social insurance supplier. Commonly, the genuine strides for utilizing a pregnancy test are very simple and can be acted in the solace of your own home. Be that as it may, the consequences of a home pregnancy test ought to consistently be affirmed with a blood test performed by your essential medicinal services supplier.

By a wide margin, the most ordinarily utilized strategy for pregnancy test is those that utilization pee to distinguish the hormone related with pregnancy. This hormone is set off when an undeveloped organism inserts in the uterine divider, yet it can likewise be created if an incipient organism erroneously embeds in the Fallopian tubes, which is known as an ectopic tubal pregnancy. There are two unique kinds of pregnancy tests. The main sort can create more precise outcomes, yet may end up being excessively untidy. A cup is given to get pee, after which the pee is gathered and an exceptional stick or other gadget is embedded in the pee. Now and again, the stick or gadget is plunged legitimately into the pee filled cup for a specific measure of time. Different occasions, a little eye dropper is given to play out a more precise variant of a similar test.

Despite the fact that this strategy for pee testing might be more precise, the gadgets intended to gather pee in mid stream are the most well known. These sticks are typically found over the counter in your neighborhood tranquilize store or market and can be finished in practically no time. Rather than a more logical task, this kind of pee based pregnancy test is favored by ladies in light of the absence of steps. Essentially hold the stick in a surge of pee for a particular measure of time—normally a couple of moments—and afterward sit tight for the outcomes. Instead of sticks that are harder to peruse, there are two or three organizations that presently have models available that have a computerized perused out framework. Likewise, there are models accessible that permit you to decide if you are pregnant much sooner than conventional locally situated tests.

For a more precise test that can recognize whether you are pregnant before a pee based test. This test must be acted in your doctor's office and will require a couple of vials of blood drawn. After the blood is drawn, tests are performed to distinguish the nearness and the measure of the hormone related with pregnancy. Remember that you ought to consistently have a blood test performed after you have gotten a positive perusing for a home pregnancy pee based test.

Morning Sickness: Causes and Cures

Morning disorder is regularly the principal indication of pregnancy, as it can begin as ahead of schedule as about fourteen days after origination. Regardless of the name, the victim can feel sick whenever of the day, in spite of the fact that as a vacant stomach is believed to be one of the triggers then mornings are a typical time for it to show up.

Only one out of every odd pregnant lady will encounter morning disorder, albeit most do somewhat, and it can differ from a sentiment of mellow sickness or nausea extending up to feeling really awful and incapable to hold any food or fluids down. The seriousness of the impacts is by all accounts most noteworthy in ladies with a past filled with headache or nausea from moving around.

It's not known precisely what causes it, however most doctors concur that the adjustments in hormone levels that pregnancy triggers are the most central point. One of the impacts of these hormones is to change the manner in which your stomach related framework works, which can prompt more elevated levels of corrosive.

Another conceivable reason is that numerous ladies experience an uplifted feeling of taste and smell while pregnant, which can aggravate sickness feel when terrible or solid scents are near.

At long last, sluggishness and stress have an impact, and most pregnant ladies are worn out and focused on a ton of the time!

Morning infection can happen over the full scope of your pregnancy, yet most ladies find that it pretty much vanishes by around 14 weeks as hormone levels in the body balance out.

There are handfuls and many conventional 'solutions' for the sentiments of queasiness, with each mother having a conclusion regarding the matter! The truth of the matter is that each lady's body is extraordinary thus no single thing will work for everybody. Notwithstanding, there are some basic things to attempt which can enable most feel to better.

As recently referenced, a vacant stomach can be a reason, so nibble nearly nothing and frequently to keep hunger under control, and save two or three rolls by your bed for on the off chance that you wake up during the night.

Sucking on an ice 3D square can help, as can bubbly beverages. New ginger is presumed to quiet the stomach, so making a tea from squashed root ginger or in any event, biting on a piece can merit an attempt.

Solutions for nausea from moving around can likewise help, so it may merit attempting the attractive wristbands you can purchase, however you ought to never take any drug while pregnant without speaking with your doctor.

Morning ailment is a characteristic piece of pregnancy and won't hurt your infant in any capacity, however in extreme cases you might be not able to hold any food or liquids down and if this proceeds with you could get dried out, which is perilous for your infant. In the event that your pee begins to turn out to be exceptionally dim in shading this is an indication that your liquid levels are excessively low, and you ought to address your birthing specialist or doctor.

At long last, when you're in an episode of morning disorder, don't stress a lot over what you're eating - getting enough vitality is a higher priority than a decent eating regimen at that point, so on the off chance that chocolate causes you to feel better, at that point take the plunge! You can generally load up on more beneficial nourishments when the infection has lessened a bit.

Pregnancy and Morning Sickness

The hardest piece of the first trimester of pregnancy is morning infection and any lady who has experienced or is experiencing it, realizes the main signs for the most part create during the month following the primary missed menstrual period, when hormone levels increment. It might go from gentle, incidental sickness to cut off, constant, weakening queasiness with episodes of spewing. Much of the time, side effects might be more regrettable in morning, yet they can strike day or night.

In spite of all advances in medication, it is extremely unlikely of foreseeing how long your morning disorder will last regardless of whether you have endured it previously. For the most part, sickness and spewing last till around 12 - 13 weeks of pregnancy. Notwithstanding, a few ladies keep on feeling sick past their 22nd week too.

Be that as it may, a few investigations show that gentle to direct affliction is an indication of a decent pregnancy, and less danger of premature delivery.

There is no basic treatment. The best strategy is home treatment. The accompanying tips do some incredible things when you wake up feeling sick as well as work when you get that nauseous inclination during the day.

Evolving what, when and the amount you eat combined with specific changes to the manner in which nourishments cooked makes a difference.

During morning or so far as that is concerned throughout the day ailment, you may find that eating five or six little suppers, as opposed to the standard three huge ones, is simpler on the body. Ensure every dinner contains some protein and starch, similar to entire wheat bread with ground cheddar and a cut of tomato, rice or wheat readiness with some effectively absorbable/light grains, squeezed orange and an entire wheat scone. Be inventive; pick low fat wellbeing nourishments you realize will entice your hunger. Abhorrences for food in light of queasiness are completely typical and reasonable.

Make an effort not to kiss dinners

Eat little, dry bites.

Try not to bounce up right away. Falsehood discreetly for some time and ask you spouse to present to you a cut of new lemon or orange or a dry, dull roll.

Maintain a strategic distance from enormous beverages, have visit little one between suppers.

Fiery, singed nourishments, and greasy food sources like rich desserts, are best kept away from.

Maintain a strategic distance from unreasonable utilization of pickles or chutney, which is wealthy in salt.

Try not to invest a lot of energy in the kitchen and stay away from the solid smell of specific nourishments when shopping.

Get ready food when feeling least sick.

Taking lemon or squeezed orange toward the beginning of the day and before dinners assuages queasiness of early pregnancy.

Suck an ice solid shape till the queasiness goes off.

Taste on cool water.

In any case, on the off chance that you have extreme, diligent queasiness and spewing, see your doctor. This not all that basic difficulty of pregnancy can prompt lack of hydration and unhealthiness, some of the time calling for recommended prescription and at times even hospitalization. In spite of the fact that medications are best maintained a strategic distance from in pregnancy, particularly in the early months, there are some that have been being used for a long time with no clear peril to the creating child.

Exercise

Since no genuinely sound eating routine would be finished without a customary exercise system we'll feel free to wrap it up with this. The idea of practicing when you're nine months pregnant may appear to be shocking at this moment, however standard exercise has really been appeared to cause both pregnancy and conveyance to go significantly more easily for both mother and infant.

The days where ladies were required to take to their beds for the term of their pregnancy are luckily long finished, and in the event that you practiced consistently before you became pregnant you will appreciate having the option to keep on doing as such until you convey. The main distinction between practicing when you're pregnant and when you're not is that you have to take significantly more consideration not to try too hard. Ladies who devour too not many calories while pregnant and practice an excessive amount of have been appeared to stunt the development of their embryo, so do everything with some restraint.

A decent rule to practicing when you're pregnant is that on the off chance that you are excessively winded to talk while you are doing it you would presumably be in an ideal situation setting it aside until after. This isn't an ideal opportunity to begin preparing for your initial five mile long distance race, however on the off chance that you consistently practice twenty to thirty minutes every day you ought to have the option to proceed with your ordinary daily schedule. Your pre-pregnancy wellness level will be the deciding variable in what you may or may not be able to while pregnant.

One factor you do need to consider is the effect of your activity schedule. While high effect practice during the initial two months (when you as a rule don't know you're pregnant) hasn't been appeared to cause issues, doing these activities as you progress places you at a higher danger of harming yourself and, conceivably, your infant. When you understand you are pregnant you ought to think about changing to a low effect, quality centered preparing routine.

Pilates, yoga, swimming and strolling are awesome for eager moms, in spite of the fact that you ought to be careful about putting an excess of strain on the stomach muscles when doing Pilates. Moving and step heart stimulating exercise are additionally awesome for helping you remain fit on the off chance that you can't stomach the idea of surrendering your fiery exercise system. Quality preparing will assist you with building up the muscles in your back, neck and legs, making hefting 20 pounds of infant around in your ninth month a lot simpler.

Attempt to abstain from whatever requires balance as you fold into your second and third trimester, since your focal point of gravity is going to move and cause you to be more abnormal than you were beforehand. Physical games that might cause stomach injury, for example, b-ball or soccer, ought to likewise be removed from the earliest starting point. Stomach injury, in any event, when unintentional, can cause unsuccessful labor anytime in the pregnancy. Your notoriety for athletic ability will stay until you can securely get back on the court.

Notwithstanding what sort of activity you decide to take an interest in while you are pregnant you are going to need to clear it with your doctor first. This is particularly evident in the event that you have not consistently practiced beforehand or you normally take an interest in exhausting exercises, for example, high effect vigorous exercise, planned swimming or running. They may suggest that you avoid a portion of the activities you recently delighted in until after you have brought forth help keep you and your baby protected and sound.

Be cautious that you don't exercise to the point of fatigue and that you don't permit yourself to get got dried out. Drink a lot of liquids when you work out, and if the warmth is extraordinary remain inside as opposed to preparing for that climb you had as a primary concern. Likewise, attempt to abstain from practicing either on a vacant stomach or just after a supper. The drop in glucose you will get from not eating may make you become mixed up and breakdown while you are working out, and working out on a full stomach when you have infant pushing on it from the opposite side could make you queasy.

When NOT to Exercise when Pregnant

In the event that you have an ailment, for example, diabetes or pre-eclamsia, you are in danger for pre-term work, you have an inept cervix or you have encountered PERM (preterm burst of the films, which implies that your water has just broken or you are releasing amniotic liquid) converse with your doctor before beginning any sort of activity normal, even a mellow one. They may suggest that you invest energy in bed rest to help keep your child securely inside you and developing for somewhat more, and practicing in this example may accomplish more mischief than anything.

Baby blues Exercise

Fortunately when you've conceived an offspring what happens next is anyone's guess. You can exercise however much you might want! The terrible news is that during the initial a month and a half to a quarter of a year of your recuperation period (longer on the off chance that you've had a cesarean) your body is as yet going to be mending itself. Trying too hard at this stage will just drag this procedure out further.

Endeavor to keep to a similar low-sway practice program you took an interest in during your pregnancy until you're feeling totally back to typical. On the off chance that anything feels awkward or you wind up getting drained stop and rest. "No agony no increase" doesn't matter when you've recently had an infant! You have an incredible remainder to work off those pregnancy pounds, so taking a few months to simply appreciate being a Mom and let yourself recuperate is entirely satisfactory.

Recall that on the off chance that you are nursing you need to ensure you're expending enough calories to accommodate your infant while you're working out. The exact opposite thing you need is for your child to begin getting malnourished, and breastfeeding consumes a mind blowing measure of calories completely all alone. You've just got an inherent, low-sway, exceptionally viable weight reduction framework. Appreciate it!

For a long time it was accepted that once a lady became pregnant she should simply relax on the love seat and lay for a considerable length of time, every single day. After various clinical examinations it was discovered that most ladies ought to do an incredible inverse.

As a rule, ladies should proceed with their everyday schedules, and in the event that they are not doing so as of now, they should start a standard day by day wellness routine.

It has been discovered that practicing during pregnancy has various valuable impacts. Practicing will give you more vitality and endurance, increment your certainty, and invigorate you the additional you requirement for conveying your infant.

A day by day wellness routine performed by the mother-to-be during pregnancy has likewise been found to create a more advantageous and more grounded child.

A special reward for those of you fearing those extended periods of youngster work is that standard exercise during pregnancy has been known to decrease the time period for this procedure by about a third. This in itself is an incredible spurring factor,

Since consistently spent in labor can appear to be an any longer timeframe.

While exercise will without a doubt assist you with acquiring all these awesome advantages, there are a few rules you ought to follow:

Continuously counsel our doctor before starting any eating regimen and additionally practice routine. This is to guarantee you will have the option to do this without making hurt yourself and your recuperating body.

Continuously begin gradually. Attempt a few exercises and don't endeavor to perform arduous activities or invest an excessive amount of energy at the rec center. Discover a few activities or exercises you like and appreciate and do them routinely, however do whatever it takes not to surpass over 30 minutes one after another. In the event that you start to feel applied or exhausted, quit practicing promptly and rest for some time. The entire reason for practicing is to help keep up great wellbeing and confidence, not harm or jeopardize yourself or your unborn.

Stay away from high heights, extraordinary stickiness, or particularly warm temperatures when working out. Getting overheated isn't gainful to you or our child, and it could really cause hurt. Be certain you drink a lot of water and keep yourself hydrated.

Screen your pulse, your breathing, and your heartbeat. This will permit you to watch your advancement and notice any restrictions you may should know about. Knowing this data and making a note of it while practicing could help your doctor in diagnosing any issues or potential risks you may confront.

While you are in your last trimester, attempt to stay away from any ricocheting, hopping, or running. These exercises can conceivably make injury you or your unborn kid.

Pregnancy causes numerous progressions for any lady, genuinely, intellectually, and inwardly. Be certain you discuss transparently with your accomplice and your doctor. Remember the entirety of your confinements and never attempt to practice more than is sensible for your phase of pregnancy.Great Activities to Do When Pregnant

Most ladies can and should practice when pregnant. Except if your pregnancy is high hazard or your doctor has requested you to remain in bed, there is no explanation in truth you can't practice while pregnant.

Studies show that there are various advantages to practicing while pregnant. You can improve your vitality levels, get your blood siphoning to your legs and improve your course, and improve your odds for an expedient recuperation.

Another motivation to work out? Mothers who worked out while pregnant for the most part had shorter and simpler works.

So what sorts of activities are a great idea to do when pregnant?

All around how about we start with those you ought to maintain a strategic distance from. You ought to abstain from setting out on any tough exercise program you are new to. Abstain from running and other jolting exercises except if you are an accomplished sprinter. And, after its all said and done you ought to talk with your doctor.

Here are some commonly acceptable and safe activities that are suggested during pregnancy:

Strolling – This is the best in general exercise for pregnant moms anyplace. It is low effect yet at the same time gets your pulse up and your blood siphoning. Strolling is normally protected all through the whole pregnancy.

Running – Running should be possible securely on the off chance that you are an accomplished jogger. You ought to decrease your running routine anyway the further along you are in your pregnancy. In the event that you can't have a discussion when running, at that point you are turning out to be excessively hard.

Swimming – This is the main exercise and the most secure exercise with regards to pregnancy. Swimming mitigates the largeness you feel from weight gain related with pregnancy. It likewise gives you ideal cardiovascular advantages and causes you feel light and invigorated.

Yoga – Yoga can assist you with keeping up your muscle tone and loosen up close tendons during pregnancy. Be certain you research a pre-natal yoga class assuming there is any chance of this happening.

Weight Preparing – Weight preparing is an extraordinary method to keep up and assemble muscle during your pregnancy. Simply remember you ought to stay away from substantial loads and weight bearing activities that expect you to lie on your back.

To be protected you ought to consistently talk with your doctor or doctor before starting any activity program. Most pregnant ladies are fine to turn out to be especially on the off chance that they've been dynamic previously.

On the off chance that you are simply beginning a program make certain to relax at first. You ought to likewise focus on practicing consistently. For the most part 30 minutes of activity 4-7 days out of each week is suggested.

One final point... make certain to keep hydrated and evade over-warming which can be perilous for you and your child. Abstain from getting your pulse a lot more than 140 and stop any activity on the off chance that you begin to feel mixed up or unsteady.

Additionally remember the significance of heating up before all movement. You'll lessen the probability of injury. Warm up after exercises will likewise enable your heart to rate come back to ordinary

Pregnancy back rub Treatment

The advanced mum-to-be is a worried individual, taking into account expanding weights of a relentless society and work place. However simultaneously, she realizes that her wellbeing is significant particularly during her pregnancy on the off chance that she needs a smooth conveyance process and the introduction of a solid upbeat infant.

This expanded mindfulness has prompted the quest for elective methodologies notwithstanding conventional wellbeing administrations. Pregnancy knead treatment is one such elective methodology. It has a lot of helpful incentive as it upgrades the capacity of muscles and joints, improves blood course and eases mental and physical weariness.

Pregnancy Back rub can be pre-birth, postnatal or during the work procedure, albeit many allude pregnancy back rub to simply pre-birth and post-natal back rub to mean back rub that happens a couple of days after conveyance.

In a pre-birth rub, the back rub is centered on diminishing pregnancy inconveniences and plans to improve the physiological and passionate prosperity of both mother and embryo. A casual mother additionally helps in the advancement of a brainy and sound hatchling. Likewise, the back rub assists with reinforcing and readies the muscles that are valuable for a characteristic conveyance process.

Numerous ladies dread a long conveyance process. However, many want one that is as normal as could be expected under the circumstances and without the utilization of epidural or some other medications. During work, rub strategies exist to help abbreviate the conveyance procedure while facilitating agony and tension.

Post-natal back rub centers around conditioning the new mother's body, decrease liquid maintenance and enables the body to be taken back to adjust and shape. It additionally assists with reviving and re-empower the new mother and consequently improve her capacity to bond with her child.

The pregnant female should in every case initially counsel her doctors in the event that she is reasonable for rub or for whatever other elective treatments that they wish to attempt. Her general goal is to accomplish a decent mental state and physical wellbeing and to have a superb birthing experience.

A Way of life

Food and exercise are significant segments of a sound pregnancy; so is the manner in which you carry on with your life.

Your way of life contemplations incorporate everything from the drugs you take, and the measure of rest you get, to the degree of stress you experience regularly.

We should take a gander at a portion of the variables you have to consider in your way of life:

Medicine, Medications and Clinical Treatment – In the event that you are taking medicine or over the counter drug, converse with your OB/GYN doctor about these meds and be certain you can keep taking them all through your pregnancy.

There might be more secure alternatives you can consider, or you may need to quit taking prescriptions, common cures, nutrients or enhancements that are not totally important to your wellbeing during this time.

Indeed, even the most widely recognized over the counter (OTC) and doctor prescribed prescriptions might be risky to take during pregnancy in light of their impact on your unborn youngster.

Try not to make suppositions. Converse with your doctor!

In the event that you are seeing a pro for a clinical issue, make certain to tell them you are pregnant with the goal that they can think about that and converse with your OB/GYN doctor if suitable.

Make sure to tell x-beam specialists and dental specialists that you are pregnant also.

Request that your doctor give you a rundown of 'safe over the counter drugs' for things like muscle strain and cerebral pain, so you will recognize what to take on the off chance that you need torment prescription, hypersensitivity medicine, and so on.

As to illicit or opiate drugs, in the event that you are pregnant and you consuming these medications (once or every now and again) you are putting your infant in danger for untimely birth, birth deformity, unsuccessful labor, learning handicap and loads of different things.

On the off chance that you are dependent on a medication your child can likewise be brought into the world dependent. Converse with your doctor about this and get help right away.

There is no an ideal opportunity to squander!

On the off chance that you have utilized medications whenever during your pregnancy, tell your doctor. Regardless of whether you quit utilizing the medication or didn't have any acquaintance with you were pregnant when you utilized it, your infant can in any case be a hazard and your doctor may need to screen your pregnancy all the more intently.

Smoking – On the off chance that you smoke and you are pregnant, find support and quit. There is no other method to state it!

Pregnant ladies who smoke lessen the dissemination to their own bodies and to their infant, and they pass nicotine and carbon monoxide through the placenta and into the child's body.

The dangers of smoking are amazing and they have critical effect on your pregnancy, including:

Premature birth

Stillborn baby

Low birth weight stillbirth

Sudden newborn child passing disorder (SIDS)

Asthma and upper respiratory issues

Do what you need to do to stop NOW!

Rest – You are going to require more rest during your pregnancy and you should get ready for that. Try not to attempt to keep awake until late to complete that report. Simply surrender to the weakness and permit yourself more rest, particularly during your first trimester when you are probably going to feel 'bone tired'.

As your baby develops it might get hard to locate an agreeable rest position. Most doctors suggest lying on your side with your knees twisted and putting a pad between your knees to take the strain off your lower back.

Lying on your side additionally makes things simpler on your heart and lungs, and the child's weight and size won't probably put focus on your veins, so your legs are more averse to expand.

Dozing on your side likewise assists with lessening the probability of varicose veins, clogging and hemorrhoids since it takes into consideration better dissemination and gives ideal blood stream to your infant and the placenta.

In the event that you rest on your LEFT SIDE, you are additionally soothing the weight the infant's weight can put on your liver and improving blood gracefully to your kidneys so they can flush poisons out of your framework.

Purchase a couple of additional pads and use them despite your good faith and under your stomach to give you more help.

Most stores convey full length 'body cushions', and even pregnancy pads that are intended to help your body and your stomach.

Backing and Ergonomics - On the off chance that you sit a great deal busy working or during a drive or in a homeroom, focus on the help you have for your back and legs during this time.

You will be sore and tired if your body isn't upheld properly.

Position your PC screen with the goal that the head of the screen is at or beneath your regular 'eye level' and lift your feet on a stool, wastebasket or seat when you can.

Enjoy a reprieve like clockwork and stroll around the workplace or down the lobby to ask your colleague an inquiry. Continue moving to diminish growing in your legs, lower legs and feet and torment in your lower back.

Stress – Stress is an unavoidable truth and it is unfortunate for everybody, except it is particularly hard on you when you are pregnant and it is challenging for your infant.

In the event that your activity, school or family life is unpleasant, if your timetable is insane or in the event that you are under a great deal of weight, you have to search for approaches to lessen the pressure.

You may need to quit working sooner on the off chance that you can't discover arrangements at work. On the off chance that your pressure originates from a long or serious drive to work, consider approaches to change that drive by working at home a couple of days seven days.

Converse with your manager and your associates and enroll their assistance during the time you are pregnant. You can give back in kind after you convey.

Let your family help you with things you can bear to assign and permit yourself to be spoiled. Be eager to release things. You don't need to vacuum each day. You can purchase great take out food every so often and request that your better half do the clothing.

Decrease the hours you work or study and attempt to get more unwinding time and rest time in your calendar.

You will be more ready for a solid conveyance in the event that you take a gander at this issue.

Dealing with your feline – This is an extraordinary opportunity to keep away from feline litter. Pregnant ladies ought NOT perfect litter boxes, on account of the danger of toxoplasmosis, spread through messy feline litter.

Your child might be conceived rashly, experience the ill effects of helpless development or even have eye or cerebrum harm on the off chance that you are presented to this poisonous substance.

What makes this issue more genuine is that you are probably going to be sans indication, while having passed toxoplasmosis to your kid who youngster would then be able to experience the ill effects of the impacts of the poison.

Watching your weight - You should (and will) put on weight during your pregnancy. The vast majority of your weight addition will be during your third trimester. It is essential to eat a reasonable eating routine and exercise so you don't put on abundance weight that may hamper your recuperation or your physical action during or after pregnancy.

As a rule, your doctor will endeavor to confine your weight addition to:

2-4 pounds complete during the main trimester

3-4 pounds for each month during the second and third trimesters

25-30 pounds for a normal absolute weight gain during pregnancy

if you were underweight before pregnancy: 28-40 pounds all out weight gain, on the off chance that you were overweight before pregnancy: 15-25 pounds all out weight gain

Your all out weight gain during pregnancy midpoints 6-8 pounds in 'infant weight', with the rest comprising of water maintenance, amniotic liquid, placental sac, and expanded bosom and uterine weight.

Obviously everybody is unique and weight gain relies upon your own circumstance, your stature and your beginning weight, also. Converse with your doctor about what is directly for you.

Studies have indicated that ladies who acquire than the absolute suggested during pregnancy, and who don't lose this weight inside a half year after birth are at high hazard for corpulence up to ten years after conveyance.

Your doctor will screen your weight gain at each visit and converse with you about any worries he may have in such manner.

Sex during pregnancy - Sex and pregnancy go connected at the hip. Be that as it may, numerous pregnant ladies regularly have inquiries regarding sex DURING pregnancy. Furthermore, in some cases pregnant ladies are humiliated to ask their doctor inquiries about this personal subject.

You might be worried about whether intercourse can cause unnatural birth cycle or represent a hazard to your unborn kid.

Assuming you have an ordinary pregnancy, there is no dread of confusions or issues coming about because of sex during pregnancy.

Obviously you ought to get some information about your own circumstance, yet the normal lady can and will engage in sexual relations very much into her third trimester.

On the off chance that you begin to get awkward in your third trimester and it is hard for you to accomplish or continue certain positions due to your physical size, you and your accomplice might need to explore different avenues regarding cushions for help, or attempt new situations to make you more agreeable.

We don't suggest sex 'toys' during pregnancy since you would prefer not to present anything unfamiliar that may have germs or microorganisms on a superficial level.

Converse with your doctor about your interests and, on the off chance that you need to do some exploration, investigate online to discover more data and answer your particular inquiries.

From your first seven day stretch of pregnancy to your last seven day stretch of pregnancy you ought to consider and take care of your eating routine, your activity and physical movement and way of life issues.

You may think that it's important to be more mindful and stop certain exercises like skydiving, yet as a rule, your pregnancy is the point at which you will feel energized, sound and Ordinary, in that you can do most anything you could do before you were pregnant.

Make sure to take great consideration of your wellbeing with the goal that your infant is brought into the world sound and your conveyance goes easily.

Most ladies report feeling solid, well and upbeat during pregnancy.

While they may encounter some distress as they progress through the phases of pregnancy, they are a long way from being invalid, and don't wish to sit in bed, or stow away in the back room as their distant grandmas would have done.

Solid Pregnancy

Conceiving an offspring will no uncertainty be one of the most mystical snapshots of your life and to guarantee that your youngster is solid and upbeat, it is significant you do everything you can to have a sound pregnancy. To support you and your infant on your way, this article has ordered various tips that are ensured to make those nine pregnancy months as well as can be expected be!

The primary thing you should do when you discover you are pregnant is to visit an obstetrician/gynecologist (OBGYN). They will give you an ultrasound to perceive how far along you are and whether your pregnancy has all the earmarks of being typical. This stage is vital and it is significant not to leave this past the point of no return.

After this, you should start to change your way of life. Keep in mind, you are done eating and practicing for yourself however for two! Initially, on the off chance that you are a smoker or a consumer, you should stop. Tobacco smoke can prompt low birth weight in children just as unnatural birth cycles and tubal pregnancies so attempt to maintain a strategic distance from recycled smoke as it isn't helpful for a solid pregnancy. The equivalent can be said for liquor and other harmful synthetic concoctions and substances, for example, paint exhaust. These things are both harming to the mother and to the pregnancy.

Another piece of changing your way of life is your eating routine during pregnancy. Try to drink a lot of water – around 6 to 8 glasses per day. It isn't beneficial to be overweight or underweight during a pregnancy however recall that you shouldn't abstain from food during pregnancy. Pregnancy isn't a chance to be stressing over your weight! Try not to skip dinners as you and your infant need however much nourishment and calories as could reasonably be expected, despite the fact that not the stuffing kind so ensure you get a parity. Low quality nourishment is extraordinary to fulfill those insane pregnancy desires however make an effort not to go over the edge!

In the event that you are stressed over weight gain during pregnancy, an extraordinary option in contrast to eating less junk food is light exercise. You might not have adored it before your pregnancy, however figure out how to cherish it now as it will pay off over the long haul by keeping your infant solid and your body fit. Light activities won't hurt your pregnancy so have a go at swimming, yoga and strolling.

An extra solid pregnancy tip that those with occupied calendars will in general overlook is the significance of rest. Make a point to get a lot of rest with the goal that you and your infant can recover and to guarantee that your resistant framework is as solid as could be expected under the circumstances. It is exhorted that you lay on your side to decrease growing and create the best flow to your baby.

To recap: abstain from harming substances, for example, nicotine and liquor, don't count calories during pregnancy, drink a lot of water, practice as much exercise as securely conceivable, and get a lot of rest! Following these pregnancy tips will verify that you have a sound pregnancy and have an upbeat and fit youngster.

Normal Pregnancy

A surge of feelings. A little stick. Will it be pink! Or then again blue? Who would it be advisable for you to tell first? What do you do now?

Pregnancy can be a magnificent encounter that is brimming with fervor and love and nervousness and pressure. There are a ton of choices to be made and you should confront the acknowledgment (regardless of whether it's your first or your twelfth) that life will never be the equivalent.

When you have the subtleties of the real conveyance, (maternity specialist or doctor), what (your infant), where (home birth, birthing center or medical clinic) and while (deciding your due date) down, you can continue ahead with ensuring that child has the most ideal start even before you conceive an offspring.

Nourishment will be one of the keys to assist you with keeping your developing child sound and safe while still in your belly. Furthermore, an additional reward will assist you with keeping up your vitality and limiting the terrible impacts of conveying your little one within you.

On the off chance that you have a hankering, humor it. On the off chance that you can't eat something, don't stress over it. The body has various requirements during this time and those necessities show themselves in different manners. It's a transitory circumstance and nothing to be worried about.

Pre-birth Nutrients – While numerous different nutrients have the essential amounts of nutrients and minerals for a normal grown-up, pre-birth nutrients have the expanded amounts of those nutrients generally significant during this valuable time. Also, some pre-birth nutrients have added the spice Ginger to help with morning ailment.

Calcium and Magnesium – These minerals are significant during pregnancy for various reasons. In the event that you need more calcium to give to your child as he shapes bones and teeth, your body will normally remunerate by pulling these basic minerals from your own teeth and hair. This is the reason numerous ladies get more cavities and have weak, dull hair during pregnancy. Furthermore, satisfactory degrees of calcium may forestall toxemia during late pregnancy. Obviously, there is the additional advantage of keeping away from abundance leg or muscle cramps, normal in pregnant ladies.

Red Raspberry – This spice is generally known as the lady's spice and can be taken all through pregnancy. It has been utilized customarily to fortify the uterus and assist ladies with conveying full-term lessening the odds of untimely birth.

5-W – This is a home grown mix Essentially's Daylight Items. Numerous moms and maternity specialist's demand they would not convey without it. 5-W (five weeks) ought to be taken during the most recent five weeks before the planned due date. This item will assist with conditioning the uterus and abbreviate the length of work.

Normal afflictions and common other options

Now and again our earnest attempts aren't sufficient and we wind up becoming ill or having different issues that should be tended to during this fragile time. Since anything that you take will likewise influence your developing child, it's ideal to utilize protected, normal choices at whatever point conceivable.

For practically the entirety of the accompanying, the best common avoidance is water. Pregnant ladies need unmistakably a greater amount of it than the normal grown-up. Be certain you have water with you wherever you proceed to drink it by the gallon.

Hypersensitivities and sinus clog – Fenugreek may help by going about as a gentle diuretic (opening the entrails to flush the aggravations and bodily fluid) and by decreasing bodily fluid discharges. A side advantage of fenugreek is that it advances lactation in nursing ladies.

Back torment – See a decent chiropractor and use rice cushions to facilitate the agony.

Bladder Diseases – Use cranberry supplements day by day as a safeguard in the event that you are inclined to bladder contaminations. Should you contract a bladder contamination during pregnancy, you could expand your measurements of cranberry and include colloidal silver, a characteristic anti-microbial. Make certain to do this at the absolute first indication of the disease as bladder contaminations that arrive at the kidneys may expand the danger of preterm work.

Colds – Echinacea is a protected elective that can be utilized during pregnancy. Taste on Echinacea tea or take a couple of cases a few times each day. Another spice that might be successful is Olive Leaf. Obviously, remember to build your nutrient C.

Clogging and hemorrhoids – This occasionally happens because of the additional iron in pre-birth nutrients. While it is commonly undependable to take a diuretic during pregnancy, there are a few things you can do. Increment magnesium. Magnesium is a characteristic muscle relaxant and will assist with loosening up the sphincter muscle that takes into account legitimate end. Increment fiber. Regularly, because of desires or explicit food abhorrences during pregnancy, ladies don't get enough fiber. Supplement if necessary. Exercise may likewise help.

A sleeping disorder – Valerian root goes about as a characteristic narcotic and might be sufficiently only to help instigate rest.

Queasiness – Ginger or peppermint tea can be useful here. Likewise attempt aloe vera juice.

This is a period of bliss yet it might take some additional quality and self discipline to adhere to your longing to remain characteristic. Simply recall, the less poisons you put into your body, the more beneficial your infant will be.

Pregnancy Ultrasound—a Passage to Your Child

Pregnancy ultrasound is a great innovation. With ultrasound, you get the opportunity to see your child even before he is an infant. There is no known hazard to you or your child from ultrasound during pregnancy.

Ultrasound machines utilize piercing sound waves (multiple times more shrill than can be heard by the human ear), communicated through the stomach divider to create a reverberation picture of your pelvis. By moving the transducer (the ultrasound transmitter) properly, various regions of life structures, alongside your child, in the pelvis can be seen during pregnancy.

In the event that it is right off the bat in your pregnancy, the ultrasound professional may utilize a thin transducer in the vagina to picture the uterus all the more without any problem. At the point when you are further along in your pregnancy, ultrasound leading gel will be put on the lower midsection for your ultrasound.

The measure of helpful data picked up from a pregnancy ultrasound assessment relies upon a few elements. For example, during fetal sweeps, the gestational age, maternal size and measure of amniotic liquid can constrain the detail of a test. During a pregnancy ultrasound assessment, you can check whether you are having twins or products, what direction the child is situated in the uterus, the area of the placenta, fetal heart and appendage movement, and the measure of amniotic liquid. Furthermore, estimation of different fetal parts can be made so as to gauge the age of your infant and to guarantee that fetal development is typical.

The most astounding pieces of the pregnancy ultrasound are seeing your little child's heartbeat, the individual hair on her head, her fast developments or kicks, and her profile. On the off chance that you need to know the sex of your infant, you can see that as well, as a rule at 18-20 weeks.

In the course of recent years, another ultrasound innovation has developed. 3D ultrasound, frequently utilized in pregnancy, really creates 3D photos of your infant. Presently, you can see precisely what he resembles before he's even conceived. Regardless of whether you know it or not, there is most likely a 3D pregnancy ultrasound center close to you.

Should A Mom-At-Home Own An Otoscope In Caring For Her Baby or Her Kids?

We are all familiar with seeing our family doctor utilizing an indicative device called an otoscope to investigate our ears when we apparently have some ear contamination, or some agony emerging from the ears.

That is all well when the doctor, as a doctor handles that task.

In any case, the inquiry is this: "Should a housewife own an otoscope and perform ear reviews herself on her child or her children?"

To address that question, I investigated the web and furthermore take a gander at criticism from many homemakers, to tap their experience and to perceive what they are doing.

The appropriate response was an overwhelmingly "YES".

Mothers at-home feel that they should play a more dynamic job in guaranteeing the soundness of their youngsters, as opposed to have this job performed exclusively by their doctors.

Mothers at-home feel engaged when they own an otoscope and can utilize it to recognize possible issues in their baby's ears, particularly when they discover their infants pulling their ear flaps or crying with some type of distress emerging from their ears.

At the point when they own an otoscope, they can utilize it promptly to investigate their baby's ears to see whether it is ruddy, which will propose an ear disease simply beginning and afterward to allude their youngsters to their pediatric or their kid authority for additional determination and treatment.

This gives them solace and genuine feelings of serenity that they can grab starting ear contaminations in the beginning phases as opposed to getting some answers concerning these ear diseases in their babies at 2 am in the medical clinic's trauma centers.

Otoscopes come in various quality and at various costs. From a twenty dollar model to a quality otoscope, for example, the Welch Allyn otoscope which can cost two or three hundred dollars, the way in to a decent otoscope is to guarantee the focal point is incredible enough to give great magnification.

I regardless of the make or model, most of mothers at-home are grateful for this creation considered an otoscope that is ending up being valuable in helping them distinguish ear contaminations quick.

Solid Travel during Pregnancy

With legitimate arranging and exhortation, travel during pregnancy isn't an issue. To guarantee that you and your baby stay solid during movement, you have to think about the phase of your pregnancy, your present state of being, and any limitations or issues you and your doctor have examined.

Likewise, converse with your doctor about visits or tests you have to plan, so you are not away during the time these are to occur. Pre-birth visits, booked ultrasound tests, glucose screening tests or Rh immunoglobulin infusions (for those whose blood classification is Rh negative).

Accepting your doctor says it is alright for you to travel, be certain you set up a total rundown of contact names and telephone numbers to take with you. In the event that you have issues during your outing and need care or consideration, human services experts or different explorers can guarantee that you get suitable consideration.

This data ought to include:

Your name, age and blood classification, and any meds you are taking, just as your medicinal services protection data. Likewise incorporate your due date, the date of your latest doctor arrangement, any hypersensitivities you may need to prescription or nourishments, and any vaccinations you may have had before movement.

Your doctor's name and contact data

Any doctor's name and telephone number you might be utilizing while you are away from home

Crisis contact data for your family (incorporate more than one contact)

Be certain you have plentiful gracefully of solution and over the counter prescriptions, and pre-birth nutrients.

Verify that your medical coverage commonwealth covers pregnancy, conveyance and different intricacies during head out and make certain to twofold check any limitations that may apply to go in unfamiliar nations.

Check the accessibility of movement protection on your aircraft, or other transporter, to be certain that you are secured in the event that you need to miss some portion of, or your whole, trip in view of pregnancy related medical issues or in the event that you acquire crisis costs during your excursion. Inquire as to whether this protection covers confusions from pregnancy and crisis transport.

Convey a wireless, particularly in case you're voyaging alone, and be certain that your PDA will work in any far off nation to which you might be voyaging.

You can design typical exercises while you are voyaging, yet comprehend that you are probably going to get drained m metal immediately when you are pregnancy, so plan for additional rest during each movement day. Clean up, use room administration, sit on the sea shore or watch an in-room film.

Eating well is significant, and your timetable is probably going to be distinctive out and about, so take nuts, dry natural product, and cheddar and wafers with you. Drink a lot of water and maintain a strategic distance from lack of hydration, particularly in the event that you are traveling to your goal.

Mull over your restroom plan. As an eager mother, you are probably going to need to utilize the restroom frequently. Try not to design excursion or travel exercises that expect you to be out in the center of no place, away from offices. Furthermore, plan additional time for 'refueling breaks' on the off chance that you are going via vehicle.

Recollect that your feet and legs are probably going to expand during pregnancy on the off chance that you are sitting for extensive stretches of time. Wear agreeable, expandable shoes and socks and raise your feet at whatever point conceivable. Get up and stroll around at whatever point you can on a plane, train or transport and on the off chance that you are going via vehicle, make certain to stroll around a piece when you stop to utilize the restroom.

In the event that you are heading out to an unfamiliar nation, you and your doctor should consider any immunizations you will require to decide if they are protected to oversee during pregnancy. Stay away from live antibodies like varicella for chicken pox, measles, mumps, and rubella. The Communities for Ailment Control (CDC) report no fetal harm from live immunizations, yet they concede that their data is restricted, so these antibodies should even now be viewed as dangerous. Immunizations for Hepatitis B, Hepatitis A, and lockjaw, are protected and suggested for pregnant ladies in danger of getting these sicknesses.

In many creating nations nearby medicinal services and the nature of accessible food and water are flawed. It is ideal to maintain a strategic distance from movement to these nations while you are pregnant.

On the off chance that you are going to a hot, damp goal, keep away from yeast contaminations by wearing lightweight, baggy garments, and cotton clothing. Change out of wet swimsuits when you can, and converse with your doctor about conveying a container of against contagious cream, just in the event that you need it.

Keep away from dangerous exercises, particularly late in pregnancy: snow skiing, water skiing, surfing, horseback riding, parasailing, scuba plunging, water slides and some more extraordinary event congregation rides. You may likewise wish to maintain a strategic distance from exceptionally hot saunas and hot tubs, as they hoist your calm past what is typical in a standard shower.

You can walk and climb at low heights, swim in quiet waters (not in overwhelming surf or rapids), ride a fixed or ordinary bicycle, practice in the lodging rec center (on the off chance that you have been accustomed to practicing previously and during your pregnancy) and run on the off chance that you ran before pregnancy. Converse with your doctor about your arranged exercises before you leave for movement or get-away.

Be brilliant! On the off chance that you begin to feel drained, overheated, mixed up or awkward, slow down, rest, enjoy a reprieve or stop what you are doing.

Travel, particularly to other time regions, can throw your eating plan off and mess more up with swelling, and acid reflux. Have a go at eating a few little dinners during the day. Try not to eat near sleep time (permit 2-3 hours to process your food). Lay down with your chest area propped on pads. Maintain a strategic distance from liquor, carbonated drinks, caffeine, chocolate, acidic nourishments (citrus natural products, tomatoes, and vinegar), and hot nourishments. Attempt to eat high-fiber nourishments to evade blockage and swell, and remain dynamic to keep your stomach related parcel moving.

Stay away from movement affliction by sitting in the passenger seat of the vehicle and keeping the window open to get a lot of outside air. In a plane, sit over the wing, and on a vessel, attempt to remain on the deck and spotlight not too far off.

You can take a stab at wearing an extraordinarily planned wristband to convey mellow electrical flow to a nerve at a needle therapy point on the underside of your wrist. Studies show that this gadget causes some pregnant ladies with morning infection and movement affliction.

In the event that you follow these proposals, you ought to have a wonderful and sound excursion.

What's more, recall, that if your doctor exhorts against movement, you are savvy to follow her/his proposal. It is ideal to put off the excursion for some other time after the infant is conceived, instead of to hazard your wellbeing and the soundness of your Baby!

Remain Solid While Working During Pregnancy

On the off chance that you are a working lady, in the event that you feel well during your pregnancy, and if your activity is one you can proceed without hazard or strain, you can most likely arrangement to work until your due date or until your work begins!

Think about your needs and choose how long you wish to function. A few ladies like to function as long as possible with the goal that they don't squander any maternity leave and can utilize a greater amount of it after their infant is conceived. Others get drained or awkward and it gets hard for them to work, particularly on the off chance that they have a difficult or distressing activity or drive. Converse with your doctor about your circumstance.

While you are working, you need to keep up your wellbeing and guarantee that your infant has a solid domain wherein to develop and create.

Here are a few hints:

A few nourishments and scents can trigger sickness during pregnancy. The sweet move you used to adore for your morning tidbit may now make your stomach agitate. Perceive these progressions and avoid these nourishments and scents so you don't aggravate your queasiness.

Keep wafers in your work area at work and use them to fight off sickness – a stomach that is unfilled or exceptionally full will mess more up.

Drink 6-8 glasses of water a day to remain hydrated. Parchedness will aggravate your morning disorder.

Get a lot of rest and permit yourself more opportunity to prepare for work toward the beginning of the day. Weakness and stress will likewise expand sickness.

You may feel tired a significant part of the time, particularly during the first and third trimesters and much more so in the wake of a difficult day at work. Take standard breaks, go for a short stroll (outside on the off chance that you can) and move around. In the event that your activity is physical, attempt to take more rest periods. Rest periods will likewise enable you to think. You might need to close your office entryway, put your feet up and close your eyes for a couple of moments during lunch or on a break.

In right on time and extremely late pregnancy you might be worn out by evening. For this situation, change your work routine on the off chance that you can with the goal that you can move the higher-vitality errands toward the beginning of the day while you are feeling new.

On the off chance that you have a requesting work, attempt to reduce responsibilities outside work and get more rest after work with the goal that you will be set up for the work day.

Ordinary exercise will enable your vitality to level too. On the off chance that you were practicing before pregnancy, keep on doing as such with direction from your doctor. On the off chance that you need to begin practicing during pregnancy converse with your doctor about what you can do to remain dynamic.

Try not to be too pleased to even consider accepting assistance at home and at work where you can. You can generally give back in kind after you and your child are on a normal timetable and you are feeling like your old self once more. Cleaning, cutting the grass, or shopping for food should be possible by others or, in the event that you have the money related fortitude, you can enlist somebody to do these things for you until you can take on these obligations once more. That way, you can get the additional rest you'll have to carry out your responsibility consistently.

Head to sleep when you are drained! You don't need to keep awake until late to complete that additional work, since you generally did previously. Your body is changing and you and your infant merit some additional rest.

Move around much of the time to facilitate the weight on your muscles and back. You may locate that standing, lifting and in any event, sitting for significant stretches of time will make you drained or sore currently, so tune in to your body. Numerous organizations flexibly an ergonomic seat for office laborers in the event that you have a note from your doctor. Seats with flexible arms and tallness, and a firm back can help. You can likewise acquire a little pad to help your lower back while you sit. Put your feet up on a container, wastebasket or stool to drop the weight from your lower back and lessen foot and leg growing.

Plan for those additional outings to the restroom. Try not to attempt to hold it!

On the off chance that you need to stand a great deal in your activity, put your foot up on a stool or box to change your position and remove the strain from your low back. Change the leg you hoist now and then to be certain you focus on the two legs for the duration of the day. Wear agreeable shoes (you may need to get a bigger size shoe when you are pregnant) and use pregnancy or bolster pantyhose to help your legs.

On the off chance that you need to lift over the span of your day, be certain your doctor approves of the weight you are lifting. You may need to quit working sooner if your activity is demanding or expects you to lift substantial weight. Make sure to lift the correct way so you don't strain your back. Your stomach muscles are now stressed so they can't assist much with lifting!

In the event that your activity is extremely upsetting, you have to rest more and may need to quit working sooner. Stress can be a lot harder on a pregnant lady and her unborn youngster.

Converse with your chief, your collaborators and others to check whether you can diminish a portion of the standard pressure. Converse with your doctor so she realizes what you are facing. She may recommend a prior leave or different choices.

Learn unwinding activities, or take a Yoga class for pregnant ladies. You can utilize this to ease pressure and unwind and you will feel vastly improved.

Be certain you converse with your doctor about the requests of your specific employment. A few occupations will expand your danger of pregnancy difficulties.

Employments that ought to be painstakingly assessed include:

Those that require truly difficult work or require a Great deal of lifting (an ongoing report found a huge relationship between truly requesting work and untimely birth. Expanded danger of low birth weight babies and maternal hypertension or toxemia)

Employments with bunches of standing or exhausting climbing or strolling (delayed remaining at work is likewise connected with expanded occurrence of untimely birth)

Occupations in harmful conditions (risky synthetics, gas, dust, exhaust, radiation, or irresistible sicknesses)

Environs with steady uproarious clamor or where machines are extremely boisterous or have bunches of vibration

Occupations that require long or extreme drives

Employments with extended periods or continuous move changes (move work and expanded degrees of business related exhaustion are likewise connected with untimely birth)

Employments in freezing or warm environs

Employments that require a great deal of adaptability or equalization

In the event that you should keep on working all through your pregnancy and your activity is high-chance, converse with your manager about taking an impermanent position somewhere else until after the infant is conceived.

Converse with your doctor or potentially your birthing specialist about what you are feeling and change your arrangements if your condition or wellbeing is being influenced by work.

The important of Nutrition

I'm Pregnant – Would it be advisable for me to Eat Diversely Now?

As a mother to-be, you're likely more careful about what you eat. Right off the bat that may be engaged around morning affliction, however over the long haul its turns into a worry to ensure that you are eating nutritiously. So what should the eating regimen of a pregnant lady resemble? Here's the way to ensure both you and your child get the essential supplements.

* Nourishments that are wealthy in protein, for example, eggs, chicken, lean meats and vegetables (for example beans, lentils, edamame, chickpeas, and so on.)

* Foods grown from the ground – new is constantly liked. Different alternatives incorporate dried, solidified, and canned. Berries are wealthy in cell reinforcements. An eating routine that incorporates a decent equalization of foods grown from the ground is liked. Underneath you will locate those recorded that are high in folic corrosive.

* Dull nourishments, for example, pasta, potatoes, bread, and rice.

* Dairy nourishments, for example, cheddar, yogurt, and milk.

* A lot of water to expel poisons from the body.

Wellsprings of Folic Corrosive

During pregnancy folic corrosive admission is significant in light of the fact that it assists with shielding an unborn child from creating neural cylinder absconds like spina bifida. Your doctor will disclose to you how much folic corrosive is suggested. Coming up next are acceptable wellsprings of folic corrosive.

* Vegetables including avocados, endives, green peas, broccoli, child carrots, ocean growth, cauliflower, parsley, spinach, Brussel sprouts, mustard greens, beets, Romaine lettuce, and asparagus.

* Vegetables including Romano beans, lentils, white beans, dark beans, edamame, kidney beans, chickpeas, and pinto beans.

* Pasta, bread, and bagels that are produced using improved wheat flour.

* Products of the soil, for example, strawberries, raspberries, kiwis, blackberries, and clementines.

* Seeds and nuts, for example, peanuts, sunflower seeds, almonds, hazelnuts, almonds, and pecans.

* Juices including pineapple juice and squeezed orange from concentrate.

* Advanced breakfast oats.

During your pregnancy, settling on solid food decisions is significant. There might be a few nourishments that don't concur with you – obviously, you ought to maintain a strategic distance from those nourishments. There are numerous decisions under each classification so pick a choice that you appreciate and that concurs with you.

Calorie tallying may not be important; in any case, weight gain is a typical worry among moms to-be so it's a smart thought to screen your weight, and to in any event know about the nourishments you are eating. Yearnings can be difficult to control and frequently changes in digestion can bring about consuming calories in an unexpected way. Settling on sound food decisions will help with weight pick up and guarantee you and infant are getting the nourishment you need.

What You Should Think About Pregnancy Nourishment

While having a child may appear as though it ought to be straightforward, it is really not as basic as we might suspect. As per research, your odds of origination are connected to complex conditions, and examination is indicating that sustenance assumes a greater job than we may have figured it out.

As of late specialists found a connection among sustenance and pregnancy. As sustenance improves, the probability of pregnancy additionally increments. On the off chance that you need to improve the probability of turning out to be pregnant you should ensure, you are eating the most advantageous eating regimen conceivable and on the off chance that you need to improve your infant's wellbeing, the equivalent applies.

Be Keen With Your Carbs

Studies show that eating an eating regimen that centers on terrible carbs improves your probability of creating Type 2 diabetes, coronary illness and stroke. On the off chance that you are attempting to get pregnant an eating regimen high in awful carbs.

In any case, on the off chance that you are attempting to get pregnant, you should realize that eating an eating routine high in basic carbs could cause your glucose and insulin creation to ascend excessively high, particularly if your digestion type is insulin safe. This can make your ovulation be perplexed, making it more hard for you to get pregnant.

Be Keen Eat Acceptable Fats

Studies have indisputably indicated that eating trans fats influence your capacity to imagine. Obviously, that doesn't mean you should remove all fat. Sound fats, for example, olive oil, coconut oil, or natural spread ought to be remembered for your eating routine as they are essential to your general wellbeing and surely critical to your pregnancy nourishment. Crude nuts, nut margarines, and avocados are additionally wellsprings of solid fats. These solid fats will cause you to feel full and stay feeling that route between your suppers. This can keep you from gorging.

Stay away from frozen yogurt and Milk

Numerous moms to-be are amazed to discover that they ought to evade dairy during pregnancy. Studies show that skim milk and low fat can impede ovulation. Not all doctors concur that you ought to keep away from dairy items during pregnancy so make certain to talk about this with your doctor.

Maintain a strategic distance from Handled Nourishments

The main beneficial thing about prepared nourishments are its snappy and modest, and it's really not as modest as you would might suspect. Handled food is stuffed loaded with additives that are unfortunate and can even put your infant in danger. They are additionally loaded up with calories that can prompt weight.

It's not unexpected to need to eat the most ideal eating regimen during pregnancy for the strength of you and your infant. Fusing these thoughts into your day by day eating will assist you with staying more advantageous for you and your infant.

What You Should Think About Your Pregnancy Diet

With regards to pregnancy nourishment getting enough protein is key all through your nine months of pregnancy. This will give you and the baby all you requirement for sound improvement to happen. Protein is a fundamental structure square of your eating plan during pregnancy since it gives all the amino acids essential for your baby's cerebrum and psychological turn of events.

Protein is additionally significant in checking craving and in night out fluctuating glucose levels. You should ensure each supper including snacks contains some protein. There is some disarray about which protein types are ideal to search out. How about we see.

Natural Eggs

Eggs have truly gone underweight in the previous barely any years. There's been worry over cholesterol, however later examination has demonstrated that these worries are unwarranted and that eggs are really a fantastic wellspring of Omega 3 unsaturated fats and protein.

Natural Meat

Meat is the most clear protein source, particularly chicken and hamburger. In any case, there have been some genuine concerns identifying with the hormones utilized in some meat, which is the reason it's ideal to change to natural meat.

Fish

There are some genuine concerns identifying with mercury in a wide range of sorts of fish. At the point when you are pregnant, these worries are much greater as they can influence the embryo. While you ought to keep away from fish that is known to be high in mercury, other fish is fine to eat, for example, shrimp, lobster, crab, anchovies, sardines, and salmon. Notwithstanding, you ought not eat close to two 6-ounce servings two times every week.

Soy Item

Pregnant ladies ought to evade soy items for two or three reasons. Soy items have a ton of additives in them, which can be perilous. You ought to maintain a strategic distance from all additives. Soy has additionally been connected to the work in progress of the sex organs of embryos, which can have long arriving at ramifications for the kid. It's ideal to decide in favor of alert and simply stay away from soy items.

Nuts

Nuts or nut spread is additionally a decent wellspring of protein particularly on the off chance that you aren't attached to meat. They are promptly accessible, advantageous, and an amazing wellspring of protein. They are additionally high in solid fats, which can help with intellectual capacity and your mental health of your baby. It will likewise assist you with feeling fuller so you are more averse to gorge and become overweight. Search for crude nuts and natural at whatever point conceivable.

There you have it – some extraordinary data on what you should think about your pregnancy diet. Presently unwind, and appreciate the time before your baby shows up.

What Not to Eat When You are Pregnant

You are pregnant – the moment you hear those words a wide range of contemplations begin going through your head, and one of the principle ones is the thing that to eat and what not to eat when you are pregnant. All things considered, you need to ensure your baby is sound and that you stay solid.

It is significant that you keep away from nourishments that high in mercury. Fish are high in protein and omega 3 unsaturated fats, however mercury is an undeniable concern, particularly for your baby. An excessive amount of mercury can possibly harm the sensory system of your baby. The FDA and EPA suggest maintaining a strategic distance from shark, swordfish, Lord mackerel, and tilefish.

The FDA and EPA state that 8 – 12 ounces of any of the accompanying fish are fine for pregnant ladies to eat. This incorporates shrimp, crab, fish, salmon, catfish, tilapia, Pollock and cod. Various doctors have their own concept of what is protected, so converse with your doctor before eating fish during your pregnancy.

A pregnant lady ought to consistently keep away from half-cooked meat, eggs and poultry. At the point when you are pregnant, you are in danger of bacterial food contamination. To forestall foodborne sickness ensures the meat you eat if totally cooked. Utilize a meat thermometer to guarantee it is cooked. You ought to consistently cook franks and prepared meats until they are steaming hot to evade diseases, for example, listeriosis. It's far and away superior on the off chance that you maintain a strategic distance from totally.

Try not to purchase crude poultry that is as of now stuffed as this can make microorganisms develop. In the event that you decide to purchase these sorts of items make, sure they are altogether cooked.

Pregnant ladies ought to maintain a strategic distance from unpasteurized milk, Brie, feta, blue cheddar, camembert, or Mexican cheddar as these can prompt foodborne sickness. Eggs ought to be sanitized and not new as there is likewise a danger of microscopic organisms.

At the point when you are not pregnant, most of these nourishments don't represent a hazard. In any case, to your unborn baby a bacterial contamination or food contamination can be perilous. Subsequently, the FDA, EPA, and most doctors suggest that you dodge any food that is viewed as high hazard. It is a smart thought to talk with your doctor, whom you trust, about what is directly for you. Eating a sound eating routine is essential to your wellbeing during your pregnancy, and to your baby's wellbeing.

Foods to Avoid During Pregnancy

Pregnancy is when most moms to be are worried about their wellbeing, and about how what they eat, will influence their unborn baby. General wellbeing offices make numerous suggestions and one of those, in certainty the most significant one, is for ladies to keep away from nourishments that have a high potential for sickness causing microscopic organisms or that are risky to the hatchling.

Here's a rundown of nourishments that general wellbeing offices suggest you abstain from during your pregnancy.

* Liquor - It is suggested that you totally quit drinking liquor during your pregnancy as it is legitimately connected to fetal liquor disorder and different conditions.

* Caffeine – You should constrain your utilization of espresso, tea or cola to close to 0-1 every day. Caffeine is connected to low birth weight just as unnatural birth cycle.

* Newly got fish – this incorporates fish, swordfish, shark, marlin, and so on, which may contain dangerous mercury levels. You should restrict your admission to 150 grams for each month. Canned white fish and tuna fish contain some mercury, so you should restrain your utilization to close to 300 grams for every week.

* Natural tea, for example, sage tea, Chamomile tea, pennyroyal, parsley tea, lobelia, coltsfoot, teas with aloe, juniper berries, comfrey, Labrador tea, buckthorn bark, and sassafras should all be abstained from during pregnancy. There are others so try to peruse the bundling before buying.

* Liver

* Non-dried shop meats – cold cuts, refrigerated pate, wieners, refrigerated smoked fish and fish, and meat spreads

* Crude fish - mollusks, shellfish and sushi. Evade smoked fish that is kept in the cooler, for example, smoked salmon.

* Crude or half-cooked eggs – this incorporates nourishments that are made with crude eggs like Caesar plate of mixed greens dressing. Crude eggs can possibly contain salmonella and in this way ought to be maintained a strategic distance from all through your pregnancy.

* Crude fledglings - particularly horse feed sprouts

* Half-cooked meat or uncommon meat, fish and poultry

* Unpasteurized juices

* Unpasteurized milk items - additionally nourishments that are produced using utilizing crude milk cheddar, particularly delicate or potentially semi-delicate cheeses. This incorporates Bria and Camembert. Every single unpasteurized cheddar can possibly be tainted with Listeria microscopic organisms, which can be destructive to your baby.

On the off chance that you are uncertain about a specific food, it is ideal to stay away from that food until you can discover data with respect to it. You should don't hesitate to get some information about any dietary concerns you may have.

More Tips of What You Ought to Eat What You Ought Not Eat During Pregnancy

From the moment you discover you are pregnant most mothers to-be have various inquiries identifying with pregnancy nourishment. What nourishments you ought to eat and which food sources should you dodge as the following nine months progress. A few nourishments are far superior totally dodged. At that point there is every one of those old spouses' stories to figure out and make sense of truth from fiction. We should attempt to rearrange things in any event a little for you in this article.

Sugar and Fake Sugars

At the point when you are pregnant, you should attempt to keep away from, shockingly better cut out, sugar and fake sugar from your eating routine. Try not to wrongly replace sugar with Sucralose, aspartame or other counterfeit sugars, which are strong synthetic concoctions with faulty wellbeing concerns. Truth be told, there influence on the embryo isn't yet settled and there is a conviction they could represent a wellbeing danger to your baby.

Sugar is answerable for various pregnancy concerns however the most troubling is the quick arrival of insulin in your body. This can bring about your pancreas missing the mark concerning having the option to carry out its responsibility appropriately, which thusly prompts an expansion in glucose levels in the body.

Regardless of whether you don't experience the ill effects of hypertension or gestational diabetes, on the off chance that you have a high glucose, it can prompt birth confusions, a huge baby messing work up, and unnecessary weight gain. On the off chance that you should utilize sugar or you need to fulfill a sweet tooth search for crude nectar, agave syrup, stevia, and so on.

Caffeine

Since caffeine invigorates the sensory system, it is critical to cut your caffeine consumption. It will likewise filter calcium, which is fundamental during pregnancy. At the point when you are drained of calcium your baby will likewise be exhausted, thus the embryo will draw on your calcium saves, which thusly will diminish your calcium more. It turns into an endless loop. Caffeine is likewise a diuretic thus there is a risk of getting got dried out. This is particularly evident on the off chance that you are experiencing morning ailment. Drinking an excessive amount of espresso can really bring about it crossing the placenta and influencing your baby.

Prepared Nourishments

Prepared nourishments contain a wide range of additives and fillers, which are not beneficial and can influence the soundness of your baby. They are commonly likewise high in sugar and sodium, which ought to be dodged. Instead of handled why not select entire and natural nourishments, which are more secure and more beneficial food decisions.

Main concern - solid food decisions lead to a more advantageous mother and baby.

Iron Rich Nourishments to Eat During Pregnancy

So you have quite recently as of late found your pregnant – salutation! That absolutely implies that life is going to change. One of the principal things you will need to consider is your eating regimen and what it is you and baby need at the present time. Fortunately, it isn't really that hard to get the right nourishment during your pregnancy similarly as long as you remain concentrated on eating food sources that are stuffed with protein and high in supplements.

Agonizing over the requirements of the baby for legitimate improvement is normal. The uplifting news is the length of you eat well, your baby will get the sustenance the individual in question needs as they draw their nourishment from you. For instance, on the off chance that you try to eat nourishments that are high in iron you won't need to stress over getting pallid. On the off chance that you have an eating regimen that is adequate in calcium, your baby will have solid teeth and bones.

Your doctor will watch out for things by drawing blood at your exams. In the event that you are deficient with regards to supplements, enhancements can be recommended and you can make changes to your eating routine. We should view the nourishments that will give you the sustenance you need during pregnancy.

Eating an even eating regimen is an extraordinary method to guarantee you are getting the supplements you need. Eat an eating regimen that is stuffed with new foods grown from the ground. Strawberries and citrus natural product are high in nutrient C. Great decisions since you need around 70 mg of nutrient C daily. Eat a lot of green verdant vegetables and vegetables to guarantee you get the 4 micrograms of folic corrosive you need every day.

Nourishments that are wealthy in iron are significant as well. It is suggested that pregnant ladies get around 27 mg of iron every day. Iron enables your platelets to take oxygen to your baby, and it is imperative to you too as it carries oxygen to your muscles so they can work appropriately. Satisfactory iron will assist with diminishing your powerlessness to stress and ailment. Great wellsprings of iron incorporate fish, chicken, and meat.

On the off chance that you as of now eat healthy, your eating regimen during pregnancy won't have to change a great deal. You ought to maintain a strategic distance from prepared nourishments, sugar, an excessive amount of fat, and white flour. What's more, obviously, you ought to consistently follow your doctor's requests with regards to sound nourishment for you and your baby.

Is Caffeine OK During Pregnancy?

In 1980 the FDA delivered a distribution that cautioned against a pregnant lady drinking caffeine refreshments. It suggested that a lady confine or even better, take out all caffeine consumption since it could be straightforwardly connected to the potential for certain birth deserts. This proposal remained steadfast even in 1994 when a survey of in excess of 200 clinical diaries led by Dr. Astrid Nehlig was distributed in the Diary of Neurotoxicology and Teratology. Be that as it may, what's the proposal today?

At present numerous doctors suggest that a pregnant lady takes in under 300 mg of caffeine day by day. This is on the grounds that reviews that are later have not demonstrated a connection among caffeine and mischief to the baby with an admission that is under 300 mg. These new logical investigations are making doctors examine the outcomes and many are changing their suggestions albeit some despite everything stay exceptionally traditionalist. This is best examined transparently with your doctor.

What Caffeine Does

Caffeine is an energizer that animates the focal sensory system. It likewise decreases your iron ingestion and it filters calcium from the body. Caffeine has a diuretic impact and it can cross the placenta and advance toward your baby. Caffeine does the accompanying once it is in your body:

* Diminishes the measure of calcium in your body

* Dries out you

* Expands your circulatory strain

* Raises your pulse

Something very similar that transpires happens to your baby with the one exemption and that will be that baby will take calcium that it needs from your bones on the off chance that it can't get it somewhere else. Caffeine has additionally been connected to meddling with typical fetal development and subsequently this prompts low birth weight and debilitated adrenal organs that can influence the capacity to adapt to pressure and to manage glucose

It is a smart thought to maintain a strategic distance from caffeine or if nothing else slice back your admission to 300 mg for each day, and a few specialists state that number ought to be close to 150 mg for every day. You may have no issue dealing with caffeine however recall that the liver of your baby is juvenile thus it can't expel the caffeine. This implies caffeine remains with your baby for 40 to 130 hours.

Basic wellsprings of caffeine include:

* Espresso - 100-200 mg for every 8 ounce

* Migraine medication - 65-130mg

* Pop - 40-75mg per can

* Tea - dark 60mg, green 40mg

* Dim Chocolate - 5-35mg per 1 ounce

* Milk Chocolate - 1-15mg per 1 ounce

Converse with your doctor about caffeine allow and follow what his/her proposals are.

Most recent Changes to Pregnancy Sustenance

As of late there has been some new exploration distributed identifying with the significance of Nutrient D all through a pregnancy. Previously, the spotlight has for the most part been on Folic Corrosive. While this is surely still significant, it appears the significance of Nutrient D has been essentially thought little of.

The investigation found that numerous pregnant ladies and the individuals who are breastfeeding are not getting adequate Nutrient D, which is connected to toxemia and gestational diabetes, alongside diminished bone thickness in babies.

The exploration likewise demonstrates that most of ladies really are Nutrient D insufficient toward the beginning of their pregnancy, on the grounds that the suggested 600 IUs is deficient. Specialists are no suggesting that pregnant ladies take in any event a 1000 IU supplement.

Another change that has been made is the proposals identifying with iodine, which is critical to mental health of the baby and the moms digestion. It is significant that pregnant ladies get enough iodine to shield their baby from impeded psychological capacity and birth abandons. A decent route for you to get iodine through your eating regimen is to utilize iodized salt and pick nourishments that are iodine rich, for example, cod, potatoes, and milk.

Choline is one more significant supplement that to date has not been focused on enough for pregnant ladies. It is significant in the advancement of the baby's mind. There have been late investigations that have indicated ladies who aren't getting enough choline through their eating regimen have an essentially higher event of tubal deformities in the early months. Great nourishments for choline incorporate lean hamburger, Brussels fledglings, cod, and eggs.

Examination likewise ventures to such an extreme as to alert pregnant ladies to maintain a strategic distance from the utilization of fake sugars, particularly for those with gestational diabetes. It is greatly improved to watch your sugar admission as opposed to utilize these substitutes. Examination coming out of Denmark shows a critical increment in pre-term conveyances in ladies who devoured only one drink a day containing aspartame sugar. While more examination is required, it positively ought to be paid attention to and numerous doctors are prescribing to utilize alert and keep away from counterfeit sugars assuming there is any chance of this happening.

Some uplifting news with regards to those delight nourishments we love, dim chocolate alongside regular cocoa have been offered the go-ahead. Late examination has indicated that these chocolates really improve vein work that is straightforwardly connected to improved cardio wellbeing. It is likewise connected to decreasing hypertension and toxemia. What an incredible motivation to ruin yourself with a little chocolate.

Notwithstanding this ongoing dietary suggestion, you ought to consistently eat an eating routine that is pressed with new products of the soil, entire grains, lean meats, and maintains a strategic distance from prepared nourishments.

Make Entire Food Nutrients Part of Your Pregnancy Diet

With regards to nourishment during pregnancy, pregnant ladies should consider adding entire food nutrients to their eating routine. This sort of nutrient enhancement is extricated from characteristic sources as opposed to being artificially built. That settles on these a superior decision during pregnancy and after labor too.

Why Moms to-be have to Take Nutrient Enhancements as A major aspect of Pregnancy Sustenance

Doubtlessly – the human body is astounding and has an unbelievable capacity to get what it needs through assets nature brings to the table. At the point when we eat a sound eating routine, we can separate the correct equalization of nutrients, fats, minerals, and vitality sources to keep the body running ideally. During pregnancy, we should be significantly more watchful to guarantee we get the supplements that the embryo requires to create both intellectually and genuinely into a solid term baby.

Lamentably, a large number of us aren't eating a solid even eating regimen and in no other time has the requirement for particular pregnancy sustenance been vital. There are various reasons why there has been such an adjustment in the manner we eat, which incorporates accommodation, ease, and accessibility of prepared nourishments. Including entire food nutrients makes it simpler to guarantee a portion of those basic aggravates that are missing from handled nourishments are gotten by mother and baby consistently. That is significant for the improvement of the kid and the mother's general wellbeing.

Why Entire Food Nutrients are better

Entire food nutrients don't utilize incorporated mixes. Or maybe, they use sources that can be found in nature. This kind of nutrient is better absorbed by the body. Sure the most ideal approach to get the supplements we need is by eating healthy – bunches of new foods grown from the ground, entire grains, and so forth.; in any case, the majority of us can't keep up that every day. This is much more significant when you are pregnant, thus entire food nutrients make a superior showing of filling that void.

The body can undoubtedly perceive these regular mixes and use them contrasted with manufactured nutrients where as much as 90% go through failing to be utilized by the body. It doesn't bode well to take these in the event that you are just going to get 10% worth. Rather, by making the entire food nutrients part of your day by day sustenance you can be certain the baby and you are getting the greatest dietary benefit. **The Effects of Caffeine and Green Tea**

The effects of caffeine and Green Tea.

Pregnant ladies would be shrewd to restrain the measure of green tea they drink during pregnancy, and should be cautious about taking any green tea supplements. Green tea is wealthy in cancer prevention agents, and has a large group of medical advantages identifying with dental wellbeing, glucose levels, cholesterol, and weight reduction. However, specialists have found, while inspecting the dynamic constituent of green tea, the epigallocatechins, or EGCG for short, that it might influence the manner in which the body utilizes folate. Folate is significant for pregnant ladies as it forestalls neural cylinder birth absconds in infants.

The issue of green tea during pregnancy is that the EGCG particles are fundamentally like a compound called methotrexate. Methotrexate can murder malignancy cells by synthetically holding with a compound in the body called chemical dihydrofolate reductase (DHFR). Sound individuals have this chemical additionally - it is a piece of what is known as the folate pathway, which is the pathway, or steps, the body takes to change supplements like folate into something that can be utilized to help its ordinary capacities.

Yet, this compound similitude implies that the EGCG in green tea likewise ties with the catalyst DHFR, and when it does this, it inactivates this chemical. At the point when this protein is inactivated, the capacity of the body to utilize folate will be influenced. How much green tea can be devoured, or exactly how much folate retention is influenced, is indistinct. Despite the fact that the examination article said that drinking 2 cups of green tea daily can stop malignancy cells (which is the thing that methotrexate is focusing) from developing.

The uplifting news on caffeine drank during pregnancy, from espresso and tea, is that a moderate sum is fine. Two investigations, one by Danish researchers who talked with in excess of 88,000 pregnant ladies, and the other by the Yale University School of Medicine, had comparable discoveries on caffeine during pregnancy.

The worries over caffeine were that it would prompt low birth weight or unnatural birth cycle. What's more, this is still valid for a high day by day admission of espresso. The Yale group found that drinking about 600mg of caffeine daily, which is around 6 cups of espresso, would decrease birth weight to levels that were clinically critical. The rate at which birth weight was diminished was set up at being 28 grams for each 100 mg, or 1 mug, of espresso every day. In any case, they accentuated this would not be huge for moderate caffeine utilization.

The Danish examination found that drinking 8 cups or a greater amount of espresso every day (this would be around 16 cups or a greater amount of tea), would expand the odds of premature delivery, or stillbirth, by 60% contrasted with ladies who didn't drink caffeine. They likewise found that moderate espresso or tea drinking didn't present critical dangers. For those drinking a large portion of a cup to 3 cups of espresso daily, the danger of fetal demise was 3% higher contrasted with non-caffeine consumers. What's more, for those drinking 4 to 7 cups of espresso daily, the hazard increments to 33%. One mug of espresso rises to around 2 cups of tea when looking at caffeine levels. The suggested measure of espresso alcoholic is up to 3 cups day by day, or 6 cups of tea, by the UK food office.

Sustenance for a Solid Mother and Baby

Being pregnant ought to be a blissful time, however for some it's an unnerving time with toxemia, pregnancy instigated hypertension, blood poisoning, and different conditions. While you will most likely be unable to abstain from having an issue during your pregnancy, there are some healthful things you can do to diminish your hazard. We should examine a portion of those eating techniques.

You ought to never be bashful about dairy items on the grounds that as a mother to be you need at any rate 4 servings or 1000-1300 mg of calcium day by day. You likewise need in any event 4000 IU's of Nutrient D3 every day.

Iron is significant during pregnancy. You have to get in any event 27 mg daily. You can expand your iron by taking an iron enhancement. Actually, your doctor may train you to do as such. The best 10 nourishments for iron are:

- Artichokes
- Beans, chick peas, lentils and soybeans
- Dull, verdant greens (i.e. spinach, collards)
- Dried natural product (i.e. prunes, raisins)
- Egg yolks
- Iron-improved oats and grains
- Liver
- Mollusks (i.e. shellfishes, clams, scallops)
- Red meat
- Turkey or chicken giblets

Pregnant ladies need in any event 70 mg of Nutrient C day by day. Nutrient C assists with warding off contamination and keep you solid. Some great wellsprings of Nutrient C include:

- Oranges
- Strawberries
- Tomatoes
- Broccoli
- Dull Verdant Greens

You likely will have enormous yearnings and yet, you should diminish your fat admission with the goal that it is close to 30 percent of your absolute day by day calorie consumption. Make a point to understand names.

Omega 3s are significant for the advancement of your baby's vision and mind.

Simple on the mayo or cheddar restricting your cholesterol to 300 mg daily.

Protein builds up each cell of your baby. You have to eat 80 to 100 grams of protein daily. In the event that you find that the smell of meat makes you debilitated, remember that you can get your protein from drinking a whey protein shake.

Being pregnant isn't simple and eating well can be a genuine test. Every so often you'll feel phenomenal, while different days eating is the farthest thing from your psyche. A solid weight gain is commonly 25 to 35 pounds. Nonetheless, in the event that you are underweight, you should increase 28 to 40 pounds and on the off chance that you are overweight, you ought to gain15 to 25 pounds.

At the point when your supplement admission isn't as well as could be expected be, you increment your danger of creating pregnancy related conditions, for example, toxemia, pregnancy hypertension, blood poisoning, and HELLP disorder.

Nourishment Rules for a Sound Pregnancy

So as to guarantee every single pregnant lady comprehend what is expected to have a solid pregnancy and sound baby, as far as nourishment, there have been some fantastic pregnancy sustenance rules set up. At the point when you are pregnant, you just need an extra 300 calories for every day. You should ensure that these are not unfilled calories, and that they are in certainty nutritious calories. How about we view a portion of those rules.

Protein

During the time you are pregnant, for your baby to develop solid; you have to have approx. 60 grams of protein consistently. Protein keeps your uterus, bosoms, and placenta solid, it produces sufficient amniotic liquid and it builds the volume of blood.

Calcium

Doctors prescribe a calcium consumption during pregnancy to run between 1200 to 1500 mg daily. Calcium is fundamental for your baby's bones, teeth, heart, and muscles to create. In the event that you aren't taking in enough calcium, your baby will draw from your own calcium holds, which implies you are at an expanded hazard for osteoporosis. Milk and milk-based items are acceptable wellsprings of calcium. On the off chance that you are lactose bigoted, there are without lactose milk items.

Iron

Iron is significant in hemoglobin creation for both you and your embryo. In the last trimester, your baby will take your body's iron stores to guarantee it isn't sickly during the initial a half year of life. You additionally lose some blood during the conveyance procedure. These are for the most part reasons why it is so imperative to build your iron admission.

While your body just needs 27 mgs of iron for every day, you really need to take 60 mg to get that 27 mg on the grounds that not all iron is retained. On the off chance that you are sickly, you should take an iron enhancement. Nutrient C enhanced nourishments will assist you with your iron assimilation. Nourishments like oranges, grapefruits, and tomato juice function admirably. Abstain from taking your iron and calcium supplements as well as nourishments simultaneously since calcium meddles with iron ingestion.

Nutrients

The prescribed increment in nutrients is 25 to 50 percent. Your folic corrosive need pairs to 400 micrograms for each day. Eating an assortment of new leafy foods, entire grains, lean meats, and so on will assist with guaranteeing you get satisfactory nutrients.

Your doctor will train you about some other nourishing needs he/she feels you may require so as to guarantee a solid pregnancy and sound baby.

The First Trimester Pregnancy Nutrition

The principal trimester can be one of extraordinary change in numerous parts of your life and that incorporates pregnancy nutrition. Numerous mothers to-be need to quickly change how they eat. The difficulty is rolling out radical improvements excessively fast can truly blowback on you and land up causing a lot of pressure. It is vastly improved to fuse changes gradually. We are going to take a gander at the four essential regions of your first trimester nutrition to kick you off on making dietary modifications without the pressure.

It would be superb in the event that we knew ahead of time that we were to get pregnant. Of course, a few pregnancies are arranged however others are definitely not. It would be incredible in light of the fact that then we could change to an entire food diet that was natural before we got pregnant. Since this won't occur time and again all the better we can do is do the switch when we realize we are pregnant.

Work towards the end of every single prepared food and however many non-natural nourishments as could be expected under the circumstances. That is on the grounds that handled nourishments alongside non-natural nourishments that contain pesticides and different poisons are straightforwardly connected to various wellbeing worries that can influence your baby. In any case, don't take a gander at this as a win big or bust circumstance. Give a valiant effort and recollect each and every change is a positive change for your baby. A decent method to begin is to expel prepared nourishments from one dinner daily and afterward make baby strides from that point.

You ought to likewise dispense with sugar, fake sugars, and caffeine from your eating regimen. Specialists concur it is ok for a pregnant lady to have 150 mg of caffeine daily with the goal that's a decent beginning stage to curtail to. Once there you can attempt to remove it totally. For anybody with a sweet tooth there are various normal sugars that you can utilize, for example, agave syrup, stevia, or crude nectar.

Morning infection can be a genuine issue during the principal trimester of your pregnancy. As your body is attempting to acclimate to hormonal changes, it very well may be somewhat overpowering attempting to manage the queasiness that isn't in every case just in the mornings. For sickness that is weakening you have to converse with your doctor. Be that as it may, there are a few things that can quiet sickness for some, including ginger, eating protein, a bunch of nuts, or wafers.

There you have it – a decent beginning to nutrition for your first trimester to keep you and baby sound.

The Second Trimester Pregnancy Nutrition

As you go into your subsequent trimester, your nutrition needs are going to change a piece. At this point you've likely gotten any sugar and caffeine addictions leveled out. At this point morning infection ought to ease. In any case, presently you'll confront new difficulties. We should take a gander at the fundamental ones you'll look in your second trimester of pregnancy.

#1 How to Manage Your Yearnings

At this point it's feasible your morning disorder has passed and you end up managing your yearnings during the subsequent trimester. A few specialists accept that these desires are indicative of a nutritional insufficiency. For instance, in the event that you long for oranges you have to expand your Nutrient C. Of course, different specialists accept that yearnings have no hidden importance and they are only that – longings. You should converse with your OB/GYN to check whether he/she figures you should make changes to your eating regimen.

#2 Get Sufficient Protein

During the second trimester of your pregnancy, your baby's psychological improvement is occurring rapidly. To support this improvement you have to give the fundamental amino acids and the best approach to do this is to build your protein consumption. Nuts, nut margarine, natural eggs, natural meats, and grass took care of hamburger are generally acceptable protein sources. Fish is likewise an amazing wellspring of protein however avoid any fish that has the potential for high mercury and don't have multiple servings every week.

#3 Managing Weight Increase

Regularly, it is during this trimester that ladies will in general put on the most weight. That is on the grounds that baby is becoming quickly. 20 to 30 pounds is viewed as a sound weight gain by most doctors. You ought to hope to pick up around 33% of that during your subsequent trimester. You do should be cautious that you are not picking up weigh excessively fast and here are a few different ways to do that.

* Cutoff your sugar admission

* Stay dynamic all through your pregnancy

* Cut back your refined carbs

* Cut back your grain utilization

* Drink a lot of water each day throughout the day

* Nibble on foods grown from the ground and disregard the refined carbs

Weight gain is normal during a solid pregnancy, yet an excess of weight gain isn't sound and can make conveyance harder. It can likewise be hard to lose. Only a couple of good judgment changes to the manner in which you eat can make it simple to get the best nutrition in your subsequent trimester.

Pregnancy Nutrition during Your Third Trimester

On the off chance that you are moving into the last stretch of your pregnancy, the third trimester, for some ladies this feels like the longest period of the pregnancy. All things considered, this is a phase that is progressively abnormal, there's a lot of development, it's an active time, you are setting up your introduction to the world arrangement, and there can be physical indications, for example, acid reflux, heartburn, and obstruction that expansion. Supplement needs are at the most appeal, as your baby significantly increases its weight and size. Protein is required for development, iron for blood and cells, and the mind requires ideal nutrition to finish the formative stage.

Zinc and magnesium are key during the third trimester. Expanding your zinc emphatically influences the phone division and DNA creation. Most ladies are lacking in zinc even before they become pregnant. The RDA is 3 mg of Zinc day by day for a pregnant lady. Great wellsprings of Zinc incorporate meat and clams have the most elevated measure of Zinc all things considered. Zinc can likewise be found in plants and grains.

Magnesium is likewise significant, not exclusively to the improvement of sound bones and muscles, yet additionally to the advancement of more than 300 substantial compounds that need Magnesium so as to work appropriately. While we numerous not ordinarily need that much Magnesium the RDA for a pregnant lady is 320 mg. In examines, elevated levels of magnesium are connected to forestalling untimely birth and a lower danger of a moderate developing embryo. A few nourishments that are high in magnesium incorporate entire grains, beans, nuts and seeds, fish, and verdant green vegetables.

During your third trimester you will become the most – truth be told, you will put on a normal of one pound for each week as the baby develops and gets greater. That is around 12 pounds in the last trimester. In the event that you've been eating a sound eating routine from the beginning and your weight, gain is on target that is spectacular! At the present time, your baby is changing over the food you eat into nutrition it can use to accommodate that fast development spray as the end approaches. At the present time little suppers all the more frequently is a superior to assist with keeping your assimilation ideal. You ought to likewise be eating nourishments that are high in fat substance, which will keep things moving easily.

It's very little longer now before you will have your baby in your arms so spend the following scarcely any months ensuring that your baby is getting all the supplements it needs – after a short time you'll be numerous pounds lighter.

Pregnancy tips you should know

We definitely realize exactly how significant it is for us to be very much fed all through our pregnancy. These nutritional tips are anything but difficult to execute and are exceptionally advantageous so why not actualize them today?

Only One Apple Daily Will Fend Asthma Off

'An apple daily fends the doctor off.' Who hasn't heard this previously? However, what many are ignorant of is that the exploration shows that eating only one apple daily all through your pregnancy will really decrease your kid's danger of creating asthma when he/she is more established. One of the investigations discovered that when moms ate apples normally all through their pregnancy these youngsters had far less wheezing and other asthmatic indications.

Eat a Banana to Decrease Growing

Edema is normal with pregnancy. In any case, the potassium that is in bananas can really assist with decreasing your swollen feet and legs. So why not go gorilla and begin eating a lot of bananas.

In the event that you need a Cheerful Baby Eat Chocolate

In 2004, Finland researchers found that eating only a limited quantity of chocolate consistently all through your pregnancy prompted having a more joyful baby. The investigation addressed 300 ladies who ate chocolate all through their pregnancy and they detailed more joyful children than their partners. Be that as it may, this doesn't give you a reason to eat chocolate unnecessarily. Recollect only a smidgen every day will fulfill your chocolate yearnings and keep your baby glad. It's a success win.

Skimmed Milk Equivalents Entire Milk

On the off chance that you have consistently drank skimmed milk and the idea of drinking the fatter, more extravagant entire milk doesn't agree with you, there is some incredible news – Skim milk has as much calcium as entire milk it simply doesn't have a similar fat substance. So you can drink with the concern of calories and appreciate the entirety of the advantages.

Coal and Mud Yearnings Mean More Iron is required

On the off chance that you have bizarre desires to eat coal or mud, it implies your presumable need more iron. Visit your OB or maternity specialist to be tried for pallor. You can expand your utilization of nourishments that contain iron or in case you're truly drained you might be given an iron enhancement.

Lady who are pregnant regularly stress and stress over whether they are eating right. A sound eating routine is an incredible beginning. These basic hints are an incredible method to add to your nutrition and they will profit both you and your baby.

Pregnancy Nutrition to Assist Control with weighting Increase

At the point when you are pregnant, you aren't simply taking into account your requirements – you should consistently remember your baby's needs too. The soundness of both you and your baby will rely upon various decisions that you will make.

Nutrition

Nutrition during your pregnancy is significant in light of the fact that you are eating for both you and your baby. To fulfill the expanded needs during pregnancy you need around 20 grams of additional protein and 300 Kcal of vitality consistently. You can without much of a stretch meet your vitality needs by eating more unpredictable sugars.

During your pregnancy, you require more vitality for the baby to develop appropriately. You additionally need more folic corrosive, Nutrient B12, and iron for creation of blood and muscles. Protein is critical to the baby's muscle and tissue advancement. You likewise need additional protein for your muscles. You will likewise require extra calcium so your baby's teeth and bones appropriately create.

Weight Increase

It's not unexpected to put on weight during pregnancy. That weight gain is the aftereffect of the heaviness of the placenta, weight of the hatchling, liquid maintenance, increment blood volume and fat. You are relied upon to pick up somewhere in the range of 25 and 35 pounds during your pregnancy. In the event that you were underweight before you gotten pregnant, at that point you are relied upon to pick up somewhere in the range of 28 and 50 pounds. In the event that you were overweight before your pregnancy, you are required to pick up somewhere in the range of 15 and 25 pounds. On the off chance that you are pregnant with twins, you should pick up somewhere in the range of 45 and 50 pounds. It's critical to have a solid eating regimen with the goal that you don't wind up putting on an excess of weight.

You will have a wide range of desires all through your pregnancy and taking care of those yearnings is alright as long as you do it with some restraint. Ordinarily these longings are for basic carbs, which are stuffed with calories that are unhelpful for us. These calories can rapidly raise the weight gain and that is not what you need so recall 'balance.'

Eating well isn't as troublesome as you would might suspect. It begins with eating a lot of new products of the soil, which are stuffed with huge amounts of supplements yet scarcely any calories. Continuously pick natural at whatever point conceivable and wash your products of the soil well to abstain from ingesting pesticides and different poisons from non-natural nourishments. Indeed, even natural can become cross-tainted. Your eating routine ought to likewise incorporate entire grains and lean meat. Settling on great food decisions will guarantee that you don't put on more weight than you should. It will likewise make it a lot simpler to lose the weight after your baby is conceived.

Pregnancy Nutrition Discount and Handled Nourishments

Pregnant ladies generally request that whether it's alright eat continued nourishments when you are looking for ideal nutrition during pregnancy. Also, the appropriate response is.... Indeed and no. On the off chance that you are concentrating on keeping your weight gain lower while keeping your baby solid, at that point disapproving of prepared nourishments is a going to be a genuine advantage to you.

On the other hand, prepared nourishments are a piece of our way of life and envisioning existence without them can be troublesome. How about we take a gander at the advantages and disadvantages of handled nourishments and entire nourishments.

Prepared nourishments offer us comfort over natural nourishments. On the off chance that you end up developing hungry while out getting doing your things done, it's brisk and simple to stop at a drive-thru eatery, request, and be on your way in minutes. Prepared food is likewise a lot less expensive than entire nourishments.

In the event that you are on a careful spending plan, at that point handled nourishments may appear the intelligent method to reasonably remain full and fulfill your longings. Truth be told, you may believe that eating meat while you are pregnant is the ideal method to ensure you get your protein at every feast without the cost of buying and getting ready lean cuts of meat.

In any case, there are numerous inconveniences to prepared nourishments including that they are stuffed with fillers, calories, and sodium. This can make you put on overabundance weight, cause liquid maintenance, lead to acid reflux or swelling, and not give the best nutrition to you and your baby. Best case scenario, they ought to be utilized as a brief timeframe arrangement sometimes.

The vast majority of us are as of now mindful of the professionals to eating an eating routine made of entire nourishments. They are higher in nutrients, minerals, protein and fiber, which are all essential to a sound fruitful pregnancy. Entire nourishments, particularly natural entire food sources, are sans synthetic, hormone free and don't contain a considerable lot of the sketchy fillers that can be unsafe to a creating hatchling. Despite the fact that these nourishments appear to be more costly, they really are better worth since you remain full for more and you get the nutritional worth.

The fundamental drawbacks incorporate expense and planning time. It can appear as though a ton of exertion to set up a supper when you can snatch something in a hurry. You truly can have the best of the two universes. Start by gradually fusing entire nourishments into your life. Perhaps the best spot to purchase entire nourishments is a nearby rancher's market where you'll discover natural organic products, vegetables, and meat that is new. Start by changing your propensities gradually. For instance, have a go at taking an apple with you alongside certain nuts when you are out getting things done or eat before you go so you aren't ravenous while out. Be imaginative.

Conclusion

Conceiving an offspring is for sure a weird and magnificent thing. It is a characteristic occasion and ought not to be viewed as an 'ailment' however you may require drug or medical procedure in certain occurrences.

In any case, with all the information doctors, maternity specialists and medical attendants have about pregnancy and birth, each mother and each youngster is unique. Each pregnancy is extraordinary and each work and conveyance is unique.

Regardless of how much examination you do and no make a difference the amount you need to control your pregnancy and conveyance, your baby consistently appears to have its very own brain with regards to how it will create and when it will show up.

Numerous new moms think back on their pregnancy and conveyance and miracle on the off chance that they could have accomplished something in an unexpected way.

Would it be a good idea for you to have picked an alternate OB/GYN doctor, pediatrician or emergency clinic? Did you go to the medical clinic in time? Would it be a good idea for you to have chosen to bosom feed as opposed to utilizing a container?

Knowing the past might be 20/20 yet you ought to comprehend that pregnancy and conveyance are presumably the last things you should attempt to control in your life.

You can and should take great consideration of yourself and your baby, yet there is a ton left to nature in this procedure.

Birth is a significant and strange procedure and regardless of how great your clinical consideration, regardless of how cautious you are, at long last, it is dependent upon nature to carry out its responsibility.

In the event that you end up stressing over these things after your baby is conceived, converse with your doctor and your family about what you are feeling.

Recall that it is entirely expected to need to do as well as can be expected for your youngster and you are probably going to be your own harshest appointed authority.

Put things in context!

For quite a bit of our cultural history children were conceived at home, or even in fields or by the roadside. Furthermore, we figured out how to convey sound youngsters who lived to a mature age.

Today, 97% of our infants are conveyed in medical clinics by OB/GYN doctors.

The best counsel we can give you for your pregnancy AND baby blues time after you bring your baby home is to be adaptable and quiet.

Try not to rush to freeze or become concerned, however be delicate to the adjustments in your body and converse with your doctor in the event that you are stressed over any side effect or issue.

Give your baby the most obvious opportunity at beginning life solid by eating right, practicing and making any important way of life changes.

We haven't had whenever to discuss work or travel, yet be brilliant when you consider how long you will keep on functioning or when/in the event that you are going to go in late pregnancy.

Try not to propel yourself, particularly if the activity you have is dangerous or demanding.

On normal you have an incredible possibility of conveyance a solid, upbeat baby so make the most of your pregnancy and get all the rest you can.

You will require it after that little dear baby enters your life!

I hope you have enjoyed this book and that it has helped you to have a little more knowledge about how to take care of your baby during pregnancy. If you liked this book, I ask you to leave me a review to help freelance writers to continue uploading more valuable content for you, our readers.

With love

FranK V. Giulepp.